JADEN

This book is dedicated to my Godson
Jaden Lane

Authored by Cheryl T Long,
Illustrated by Mileidy Fernandez

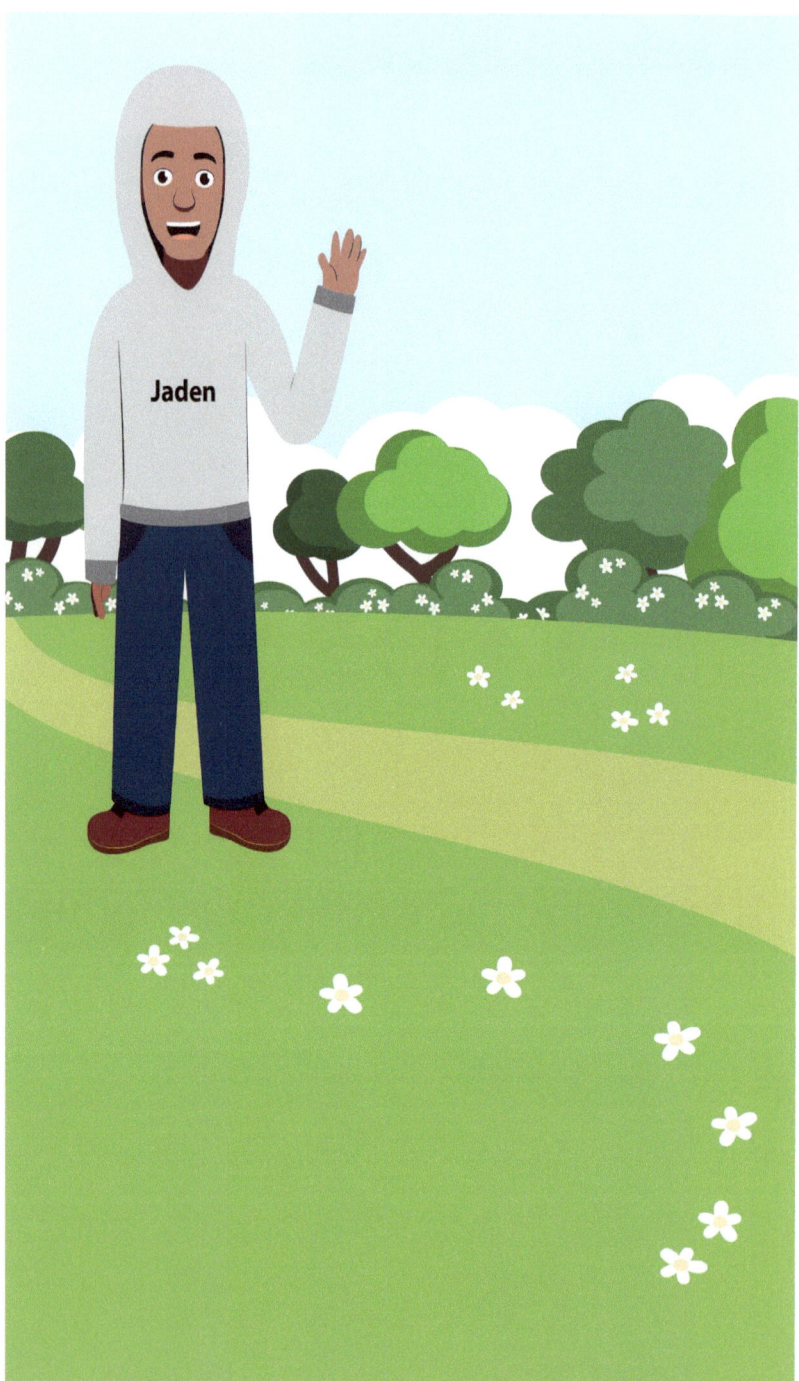

Hello my name is Jaden I'm six years old. I have a disease in my body called Sickle Cell Amemia.

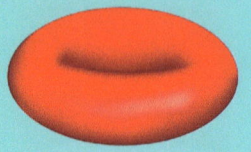

Normal red blood cell

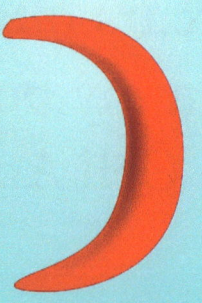

Sickled red blood cell

Sickle Cell Anemia is a blood disorder that affects the red blood cells in the body.

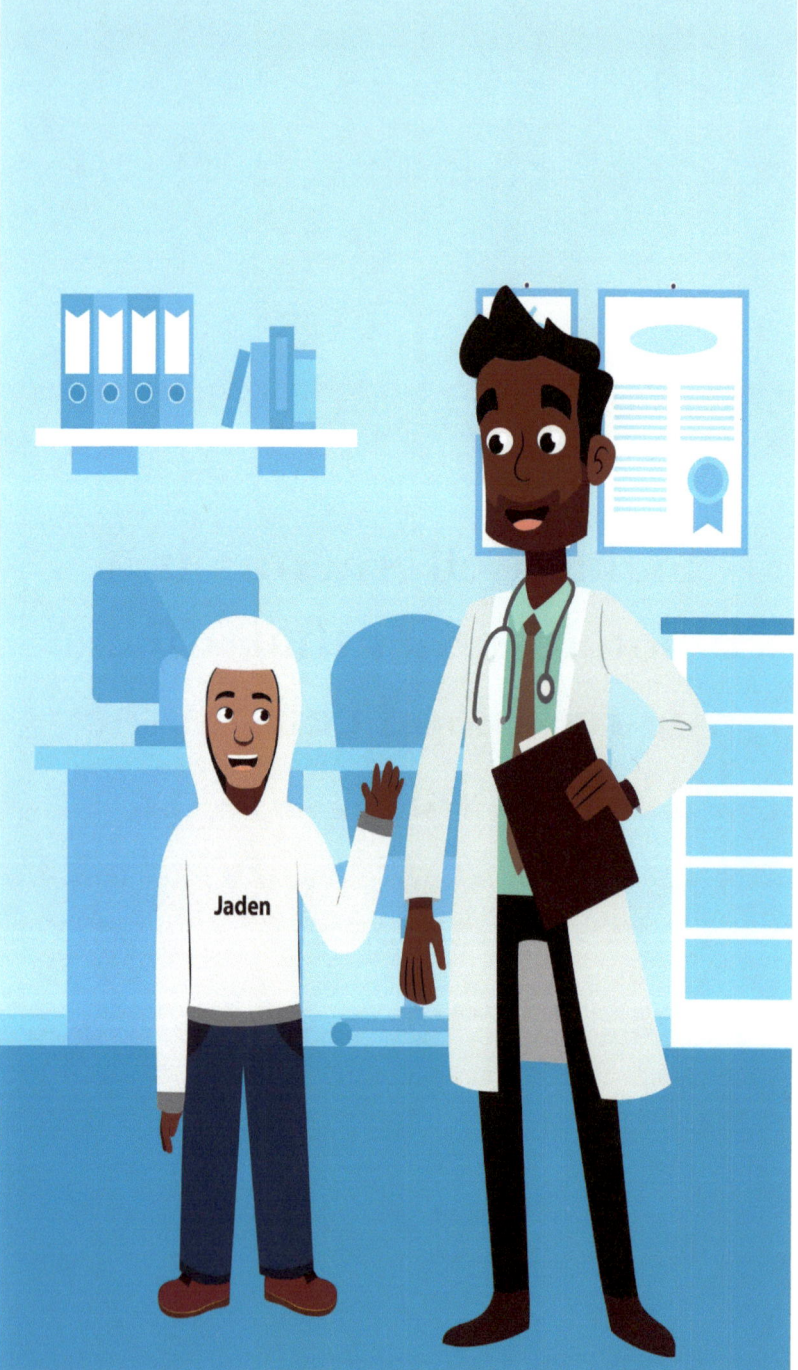

My doctor is Doctor Ken. I like him very much. He is very cool. He sometimes tell me stories about when he was small like me.

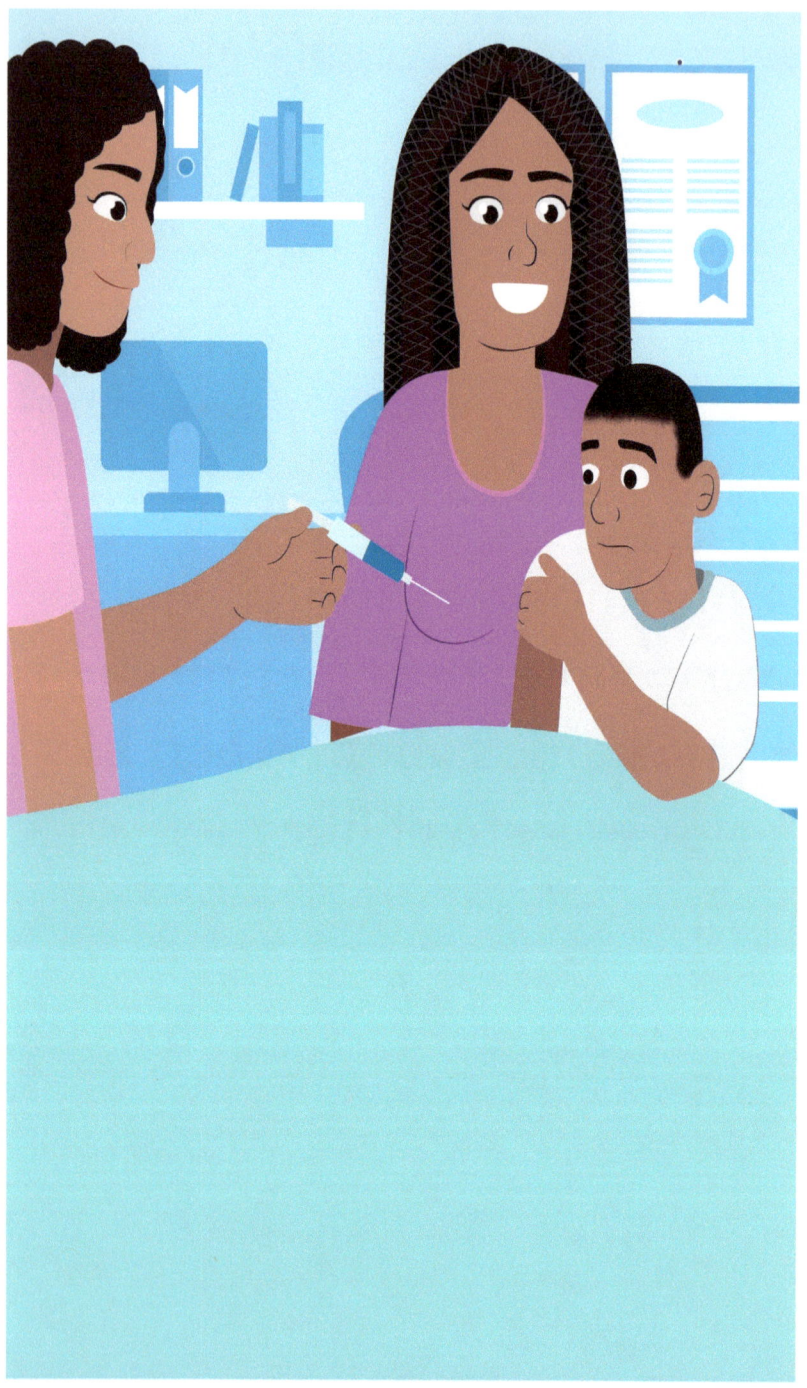

I hate going to the hospital.
But mom says I need to go.
At the hospital the nurses
always prick my skin with
the needle to give me blood.

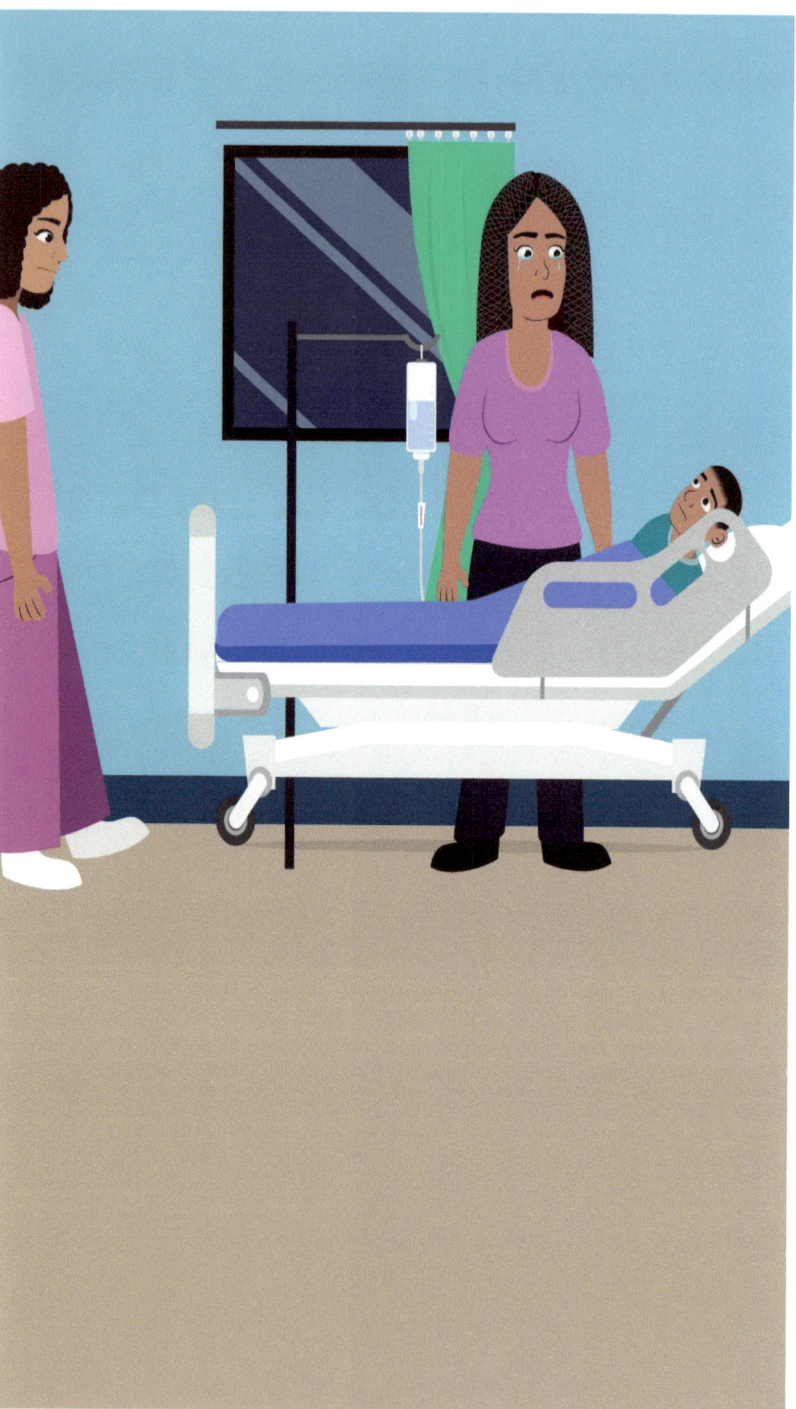

My mom comes to my bedside and hug me. Tears begin to flow down her face. "Mom don't cry I will be okay"

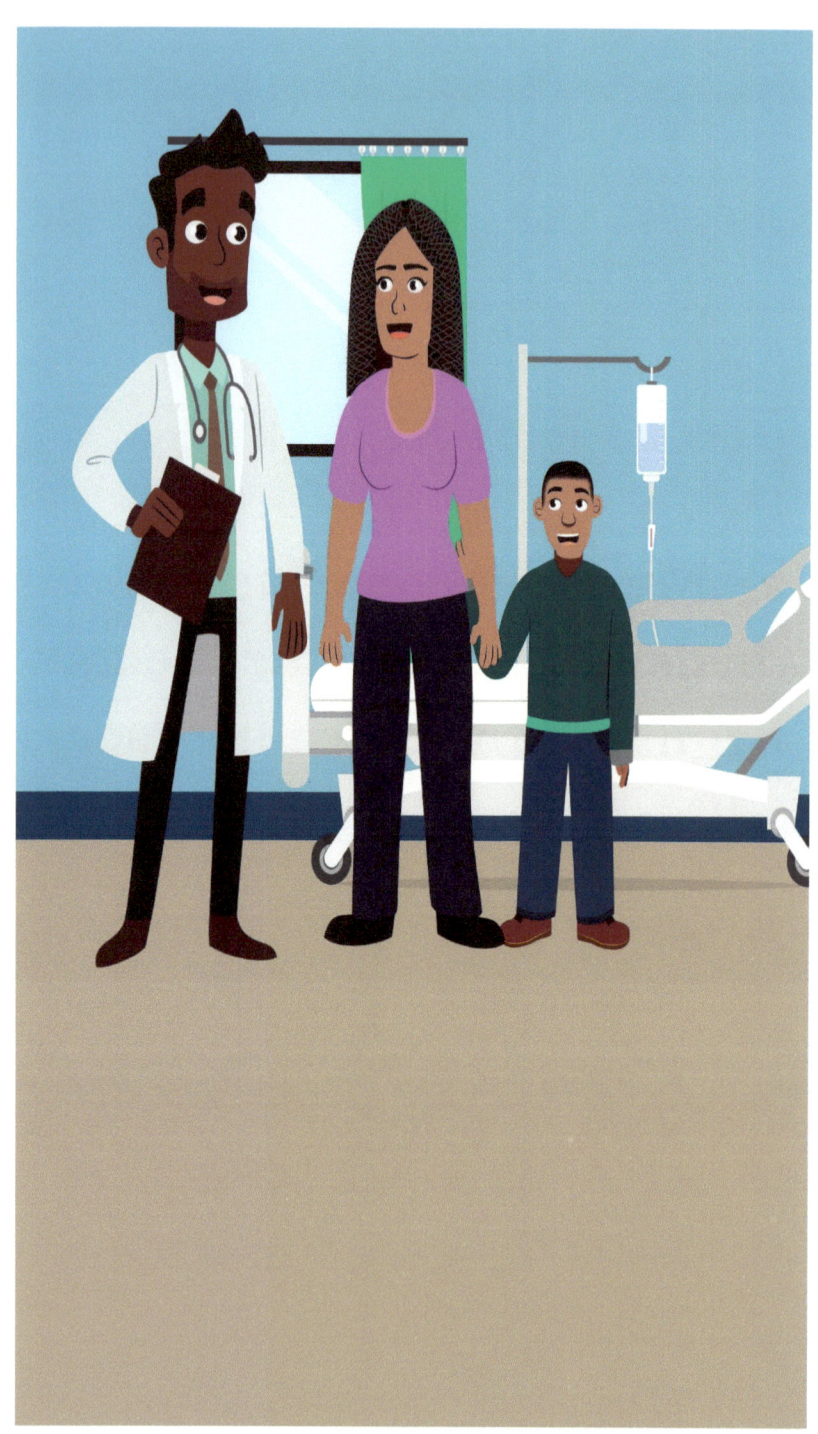

Doctor Ken explain my present condition to mom.
I don't understand all the things he said,
but he high fives my hand and says
"my buddy will be just fine."

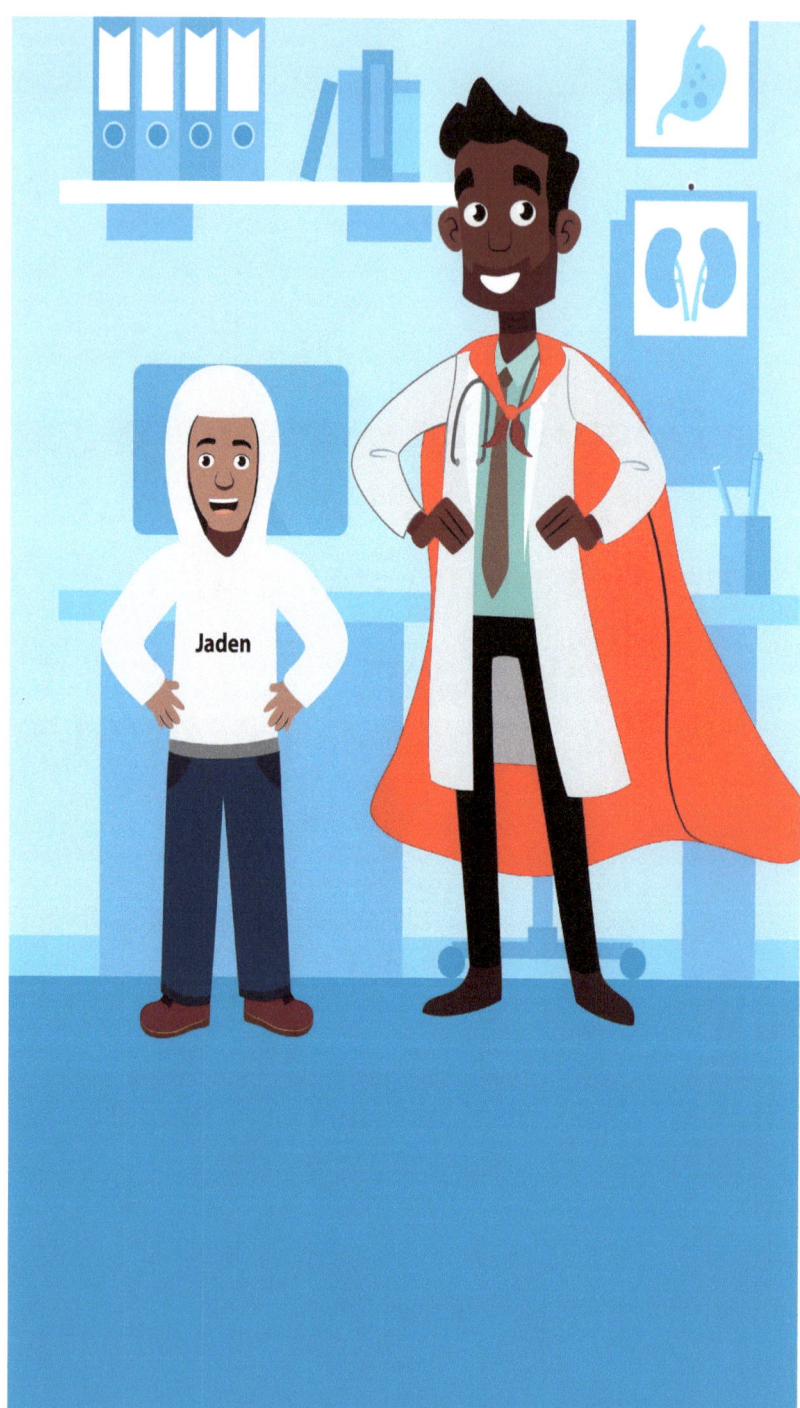

Doctor Ken wanted to be a superhero when he was small. And now he is. He's saving kids like me from dying.
I want to be a superhero too.

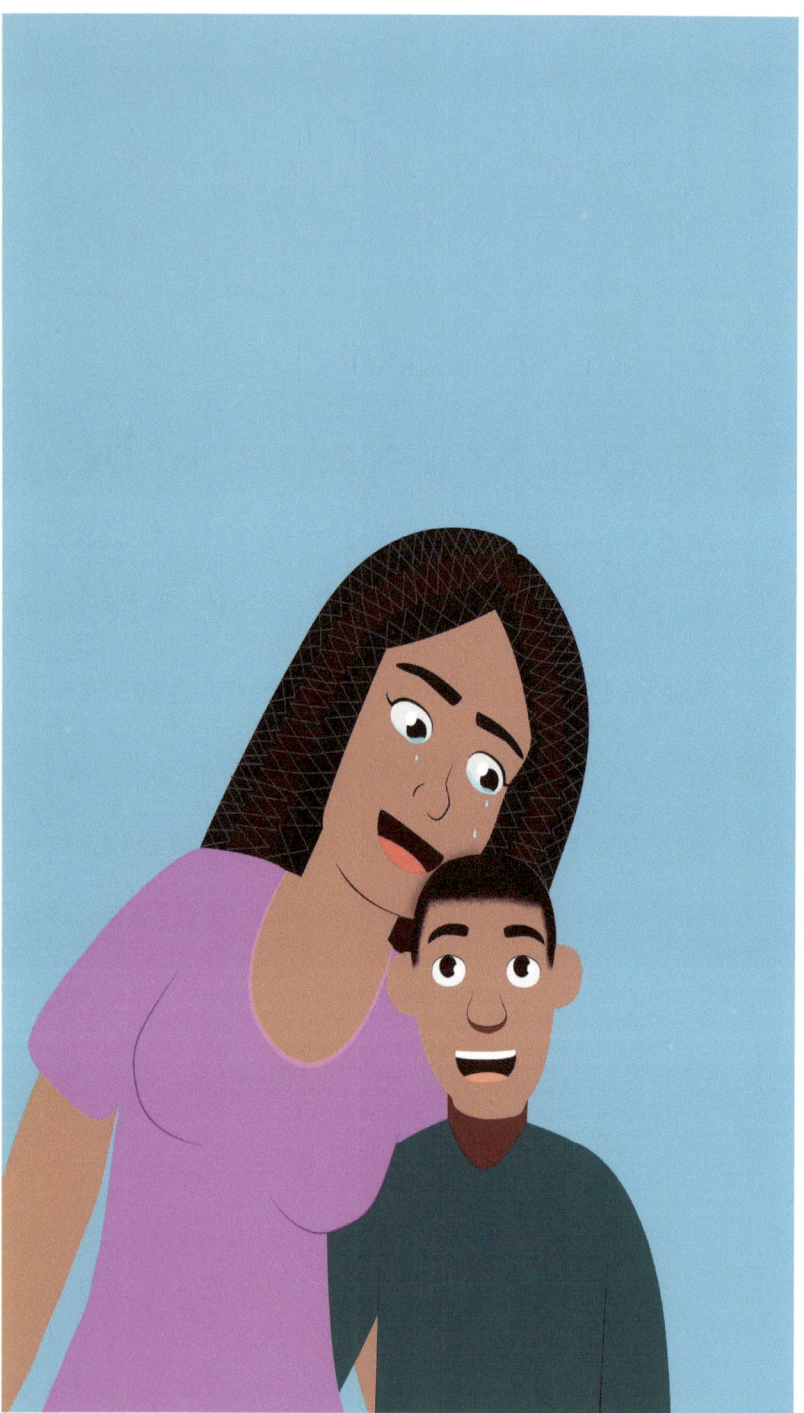

My mom is happy to hear what Doctor Ken said she started crying again. "Did you hear what Doctor Ken said baby you'll be better soon"

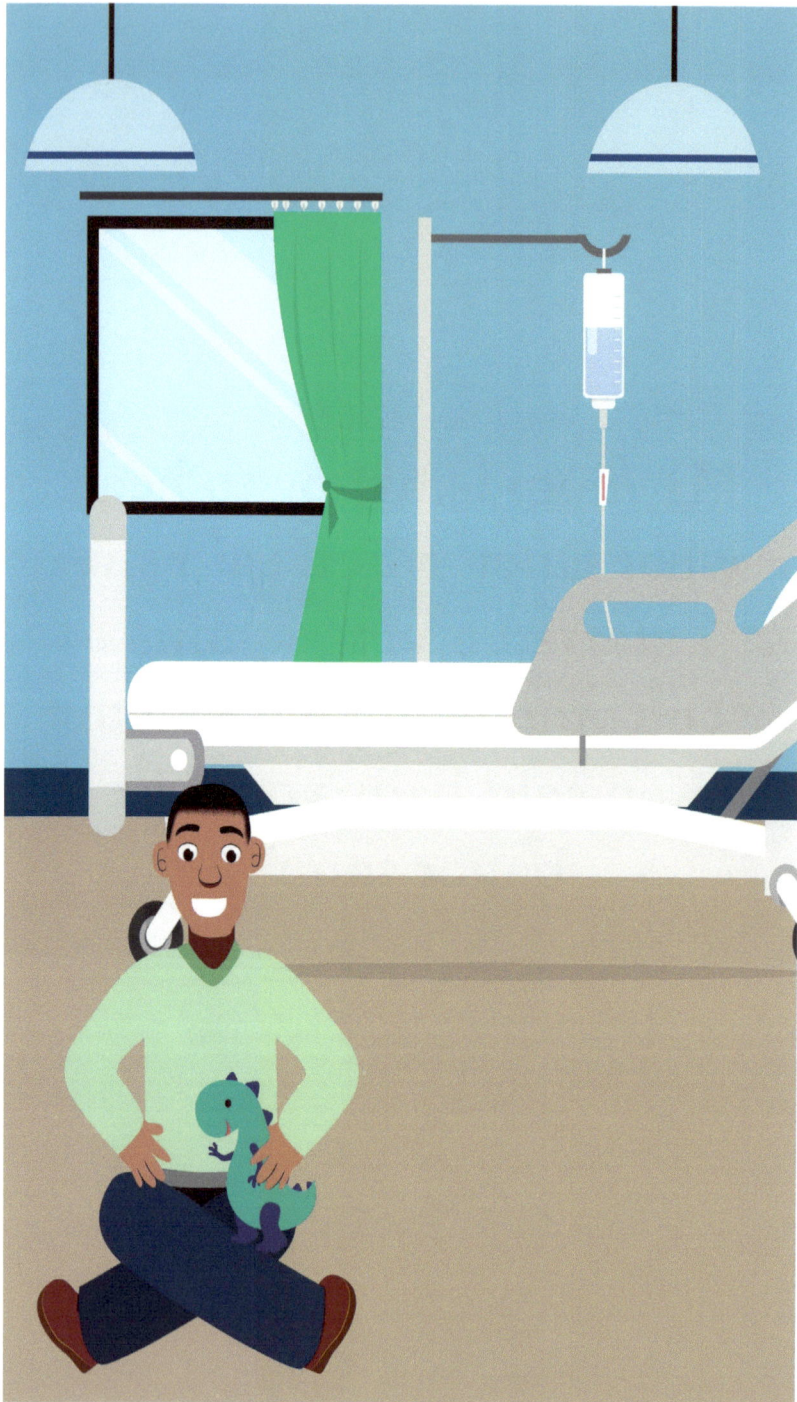

My mom brought
me a dinosaur
because I'm so brave.
I'll named him
Ken, after Doctor Ken.

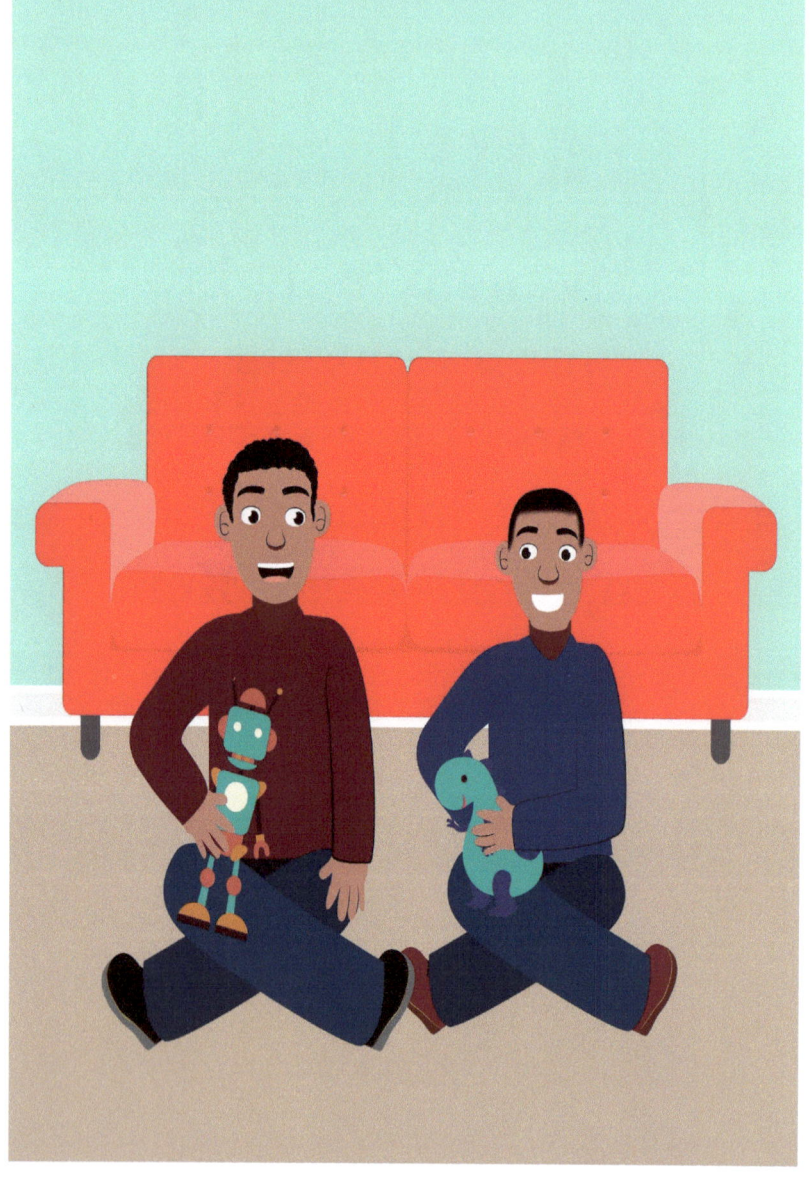

This is my cousin Adrian and he is six years old like me. Whenever I'm not in the hospital Adrian comes over to play with me. Sometimes he treats me like a girl because he's afraid he'll hurt me. But I'm a tough guy I say to him.

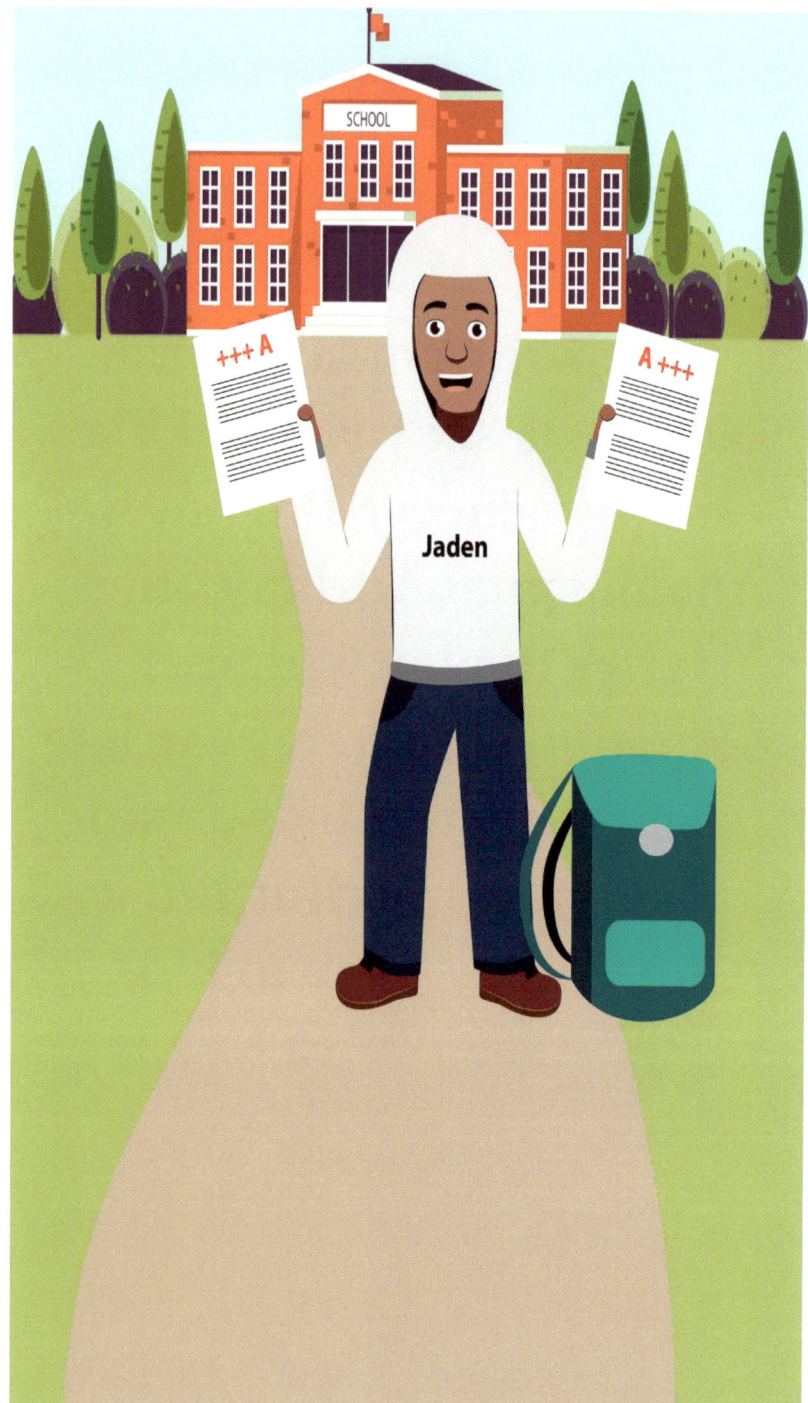

When I'm not in the hospital, I'm at school getting good grades. Look at my grades they are all A's. I love school a lot!

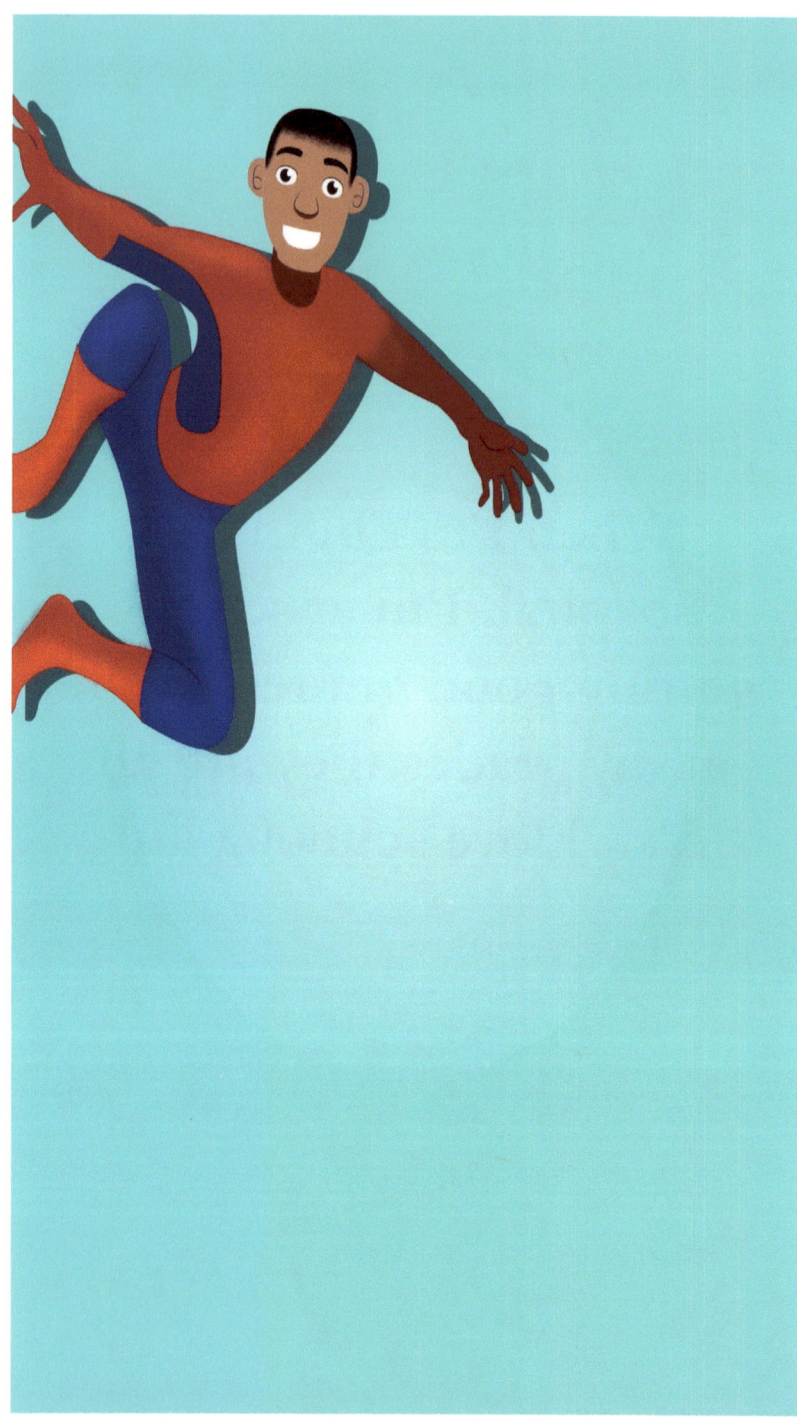

www.ingramcontent.com/pod-product-compliance
Lightning Source LLC
Chambersburg PA
CBHW040307220526
45473CB00002B/602